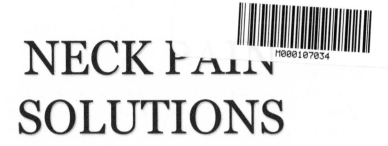

NECK PAIN SOLUTIONS

EXERCISES FOR RELIEF OF NECK PAIN, ARM PAIN, AND HEADACHES

JEREMY SUTTON

AND

MARK GREEN

OUR FREE GIFT TO YOU

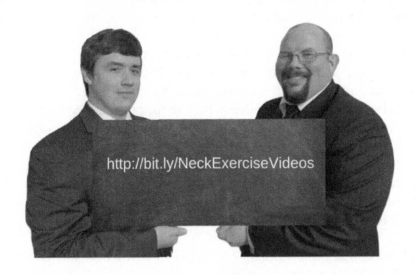

This book contains many great exercises for people with neck pain. We have provided images and detailed descriptions to help our readers perform the exercises correctly.

We also understand that it can be difficult to learn a new exercise from pictures and text alone. Therefore, we are giving you FREE access to videos of each exercise to help ensure that you are performing the exercises correctly.

To access these videos, visit http://bit.ly/NeckExerciseVideos.

HEALTH ADVICE DISCLAIMER

We made every effort to make sure we accurately represented injury advice and prognosis given in this book. However, everything in this book is based on typical representations of those injuries and their prognosis that we commonly see in physical therapy. This information is not intended to represent every individual and potential injury. Every person and injury can be completely different and varied in so many ways. Recovery from injuries can also be completely varied depending on the person, medical history, posture, activity level, motivation, and many other factors. We CANNOT give 100% complete accurate diagnosis and prognosis without a thorough physical therapy evaluation. The advice given here for management of neck pain cannot be deemed fully accurate without an evaluation from a physical therapist or other primary care provider.

Please contact your primary care provider if you have any concerns about performing anything in this book.

Contents

Introduction: How to Use This Book

The goal of this book is to help you immediately take action to regain control over your neck pain.

Have you ever spent hours reading a 200-page book, only to ask yourself at the end: "But how do I use it?" You were probably more confused and more frustrated than when you started the book…and you still had neck pain!

This book is different! Within twenty minutes, you will be able to start an exercise program that allows you to take control of your neck pain.

Use this simple chart to get the most from the exercises in this book:

What Hurts?	Read This!
Neck Pain Only	**Chapter 1**: Foundational Exercises
Neck Pain and Headaches	**Chapter 1**: Foundational Exercises **Chapter 2**: Headache Help
Neck Pain and Arm Pain	**Chapter 1**: Foundational Exercises **Chapter 3**: Arm Pain Relief
Neck Pain, Arm Pain, and Headaches	**Chapter 1**: Foundational Exercises **Chapter 2**: Headache Help **Chapter 3**: Arm Pain Relief

As you can see, every reader should follow the program outlined in Chapter 1. Depending on your specific needs, you might also benefit from the exercises in Chapter 2 and/or Chapter 3.

The remaining chapters will help you understand how to manage your neck pain during specific situations. Chapter 4 contains three very useful exercises for reducing your neck pain during a flare-up, such as when you awake with severe pain. Chapter 5 covers several helpful tips for getting more restful sleep and for sitting with less neck pain. Chapter 6 provides answers to the most common questions from people with neck pain.

Let's get started with Chapter 1: Foundational Exercises for Neck Pain!

Foundational Exercises for Neck Pain

"What are the best exercises for neck pain?" That's the question that every person with neck pain wants to have answered. While it's impossible to create a list of exercises that help every person with neck pain, it **is** possible to show you the exercises that help **most** people with neck pain.

This chapter has eight of the top exercises for stretching and strengthening the muscles of your neck and shoulders. Many research studies have shown that the combination of stretching and strengthening provides great results for people with neck pain.[1-2]

First, let's talk about stretching your neck to help relax the muscles that could be causing you to have neck pain. There are several benefits of stretching that we will briefly discuss. Stretching improves flexibility of your muscles to help you move better.[3] It increases circulation to the muscles, which improves blood flow to those muscles.[4-5] Stretching is also good for relieving the tension we hold in our neck and shoulders from stress.

The first three exercises will cover the most important stretches to help relieve your neck pain. These stretches should be held for 20-30 seconds and repeated 3-5 times per side.

Foundational Exercises for Neck Pain

The last five exercises are for improving the strength of your neck and shoulder muscles. Strengthening your neck and shoulders plays an important role in preventing or decreasing neck pain. All five of these strengthening exercises can be done at home without much equipment.

This book isn't aimed at the performance athlete, which is why the reps for these strengthening exercises are set at 10-15 with 2-3 sets each. This is to decrease existing neck pain or to lower the risk of the pain coming back. It would be totally appropriate and would build more strength to progressively use heavier weights or stronger bands to further strengthen these muscles once your pain is gone.

You can tell if you are doing the correct number of reps with an exercise if the last 2-3 reps are difficult to complete. This is how you should determine if you are doing the appropriate number of strengthening exercises rather than a standard "3 sets of 10."

You could feel muscle soreness and some burning in the muscles just as you would after performing any exercise for the first time or manual work. You could be sore for up to 2-3 days after performing the exercises.

However, at no time should you have sharp or shooting pain, numbness, or tingling that radiates into your upper back or down your arms. If you experience any of these symptoms, **stop immediately** and seek further medical care before resuming them.

Now let's get to the exercises!

Exercise 1: Upper Trapezius Stretch

The first muscle to stretch will be the upper trapezius muscle. This muscle runs from the collar bone, the shoulder, and the shoulder blade to the bones in the neck and the bottom of the head. It turns and bends the head, and it also helps hold the head up. Many people will say this muscle is where they hold all of their tension.

Sit or stand up straight while looking forward. Take your right hand and reach up and over your head. Rest your right hand on the top of your head with the fingers over the side of your head. Gently pull your head to the right, bringing your right ear towards your right shoulder. Hold this stretch for 20-30 seconds.

Return your head to a straight position after each stretch. Rest for a few seconds and repeat the stretch for a total of 3-5 times on the right side. Repeat the stretch on the other side.

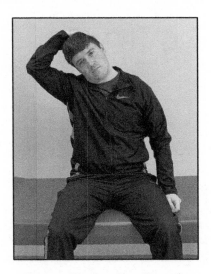

Upper Trapezius Stretch

Exercise 2: Levator Scapulae Stretch

The levator scapulae muscles run from the shoulder blade to the sides of the first 4 bones of the neck on either side. This muscle helps the head look up or tilt sideways and moves the shoulder blades.

Sit or stand up straight while looking forward. Turn your head to the right and look down towards your armpit. Think about sniffing under your arm for deodorant. Take your right hand and rest it on the top of your head with the fingers over the back of your head. Gently pull your head down, pulling your nose towards your right armpit. Hold this stretch for 20-30 seconds.

Return your head to a straight position after each stretch. Rest for a few seconds and repeat the stretch for a total of 3-5 times. Repeat the stretch on the other side.

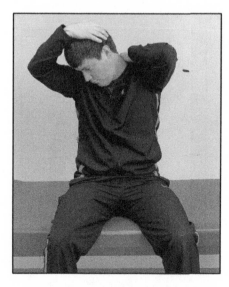

Levator Scapulae Stretch

Exercise 3: Pectoralis Major and Minor Stretch

The pectoralis major and minor are the chest muscles. They help move the shoulder and the shoulder blade during arm movement. When they are tight, these muscles can pull your shoulders forward and put some stress on your neck.

Find an empty corner in your house and face the corner. Put your feet together and place them about 12 inches from the corner. Bring both of your arms up with your elbows about shoulder height (or whatever height is comfortable). Put your hands on the wall on either side of the corner and rest your elbows on the wall. Lean into the corner, moving your nose closer to the corner. Keep your knees and back straight. Pretend there is a broom-stick from your feet to your head, and don't bend forward. Just lean.

You should feel a gentle stretch in the front of your chest and arms. Hold for 20-30 seconds. Return to standing position. Rest a few seconds and repeat 3-5 times.

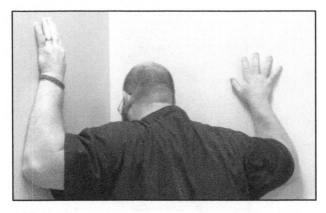

Pectoralis Major and Minor Stretch

Exercise 4: Shoulder Shrugs

Shoulder shrugs work the upper trapezius, the same muscle that you stretch with Exercise 1. Getting this muscle to move in several ways can help decrease tension in the neck.

Shrugs can be performed sitting or standing with an upright posture. Shrug your shoulders up towards your ears in a straight line. Do not roll your shoulders.

Hold this position for 3 seconds also. Relax your shoulders by slowly lowering your arms back to the starting position. Repeat 10-15 times and do 2-3 sets.

As your pain improves, you can also strengthen the upper trapezius muscle by adding a dumbbell to each hand. Don't be afraid to use weights that are 10-20 pounds or even heavier. Start light and build up slowly as you get stronger.

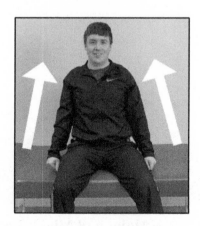

Shoulder Shrugs

Exercise 5: Shoulder Blade Squeezes

Shoulder blade squeezes work the middle trapezius and rhomboid muscles that are in the upper part of your back between your shoulder blades. These muscles coordinate with other neck and shoulder muscles to help your shoulder blades move properly when you move your arms.

This exercise can be performed sitting, standing, or lying on your back. To keep things simple, try this exercise while sitting. Sit upright with your arms at your sides. Squeeze your shoulder blades together like you are trying to pinch a piece of paper between them. Sometimes it helps to think about pulling your shoulder blades back and down rather than straight back.

Hold this position for 3 seconds and relax. Repeat 10-15 times and do 2-3 sets.

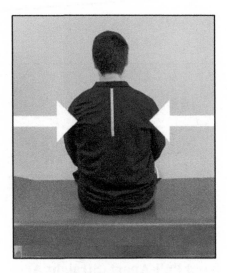

Shoulder Blade Squeezes

Exercise 6: Band Pull-Apart (Straight Arms)

This exercise works the same muscles as the shoulder blade squeezes, and it strengthens the back of the shoulders also. Like the name says, this exercise uses an exercise band that can be purchased at sporting goods stores or online. You can also modify the exercise to use dumbbells or even soup cans.

Start with your arms held straight in front of you at shoulder height. Keep your elbows locked straight. Start with your hands together, palms facing down or each other. Slowly move your hands away from each other until they are out to your side. It is okay if you can't move your arms completely to your side. Just do it at your comfort level.

Pause at the end of your comfortable range of motion for one second and return to the starting position. Perform this exercise 10-15 times and do 2-3 sets.

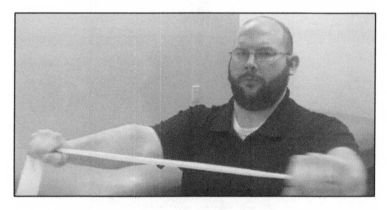

Band Pull-Apart (Straight Arms)

If you don't have an exercise band, you can work the same muscles by using dumbbells or household items such as soup cans. The specific object you use is not important. Just make sure that it provides enough resistance to make the exercise challenging.

Lie face down on your bed with one arm hanging down toward the floor with a weight in that hand. In this starting position, the back of your hand will face away from your body and your palm will face toward you.

Slowly lift your arm out to the side until it is parallel to the floor. If you cannot lift that high, that is okay. Try to raise it higher over time until you can reach the correct height. At this end position, the back of your hand will face toward the ceiling.

Pause at the end of your comfortable range of motion for one second and return to the starting position. Perform this exercise 10-15 times and do 2-3 sets.

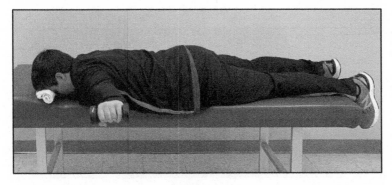

Modification for Band Pull-Apart (Straight Arms)

Exercise 7: Band Pull-Apart (Bent Arms)

This exercise is similar to Exercise 6. You will probably feel this one in the back and side of your shoulders.

Sit or stand with your upper arms tucked into your sides. Bend your elbows up to a 90-degree angle or like an "L." Grab the exercise band with both hands and wrap the band lightly around your hands until there is slight tension on the band.

Move your hands apart by rotating your shoulders outward, stopping at your comfort level. Think about trying to pull the band apart while keeping your upper arms tucked into your sides. Pause at the end of your comfortable range of motion for one second and return to the starting position. Perform this exercise 10-15 times and do 2-3 sets.

You will find that this exercise is more difficult than the previous exercise. Be sure to keep your upper arms tucked in. This will decrease the range of motion of the exercise, but it will make your muscles work harder.

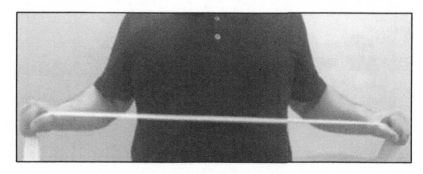

Band Pull-Apart (Bent Arms)

Like Exercise 6, you can use dumbbells or soup cans to work the same muscles if you don't have a band. Again, the specific object you use is not important; just make sure that it provides enough resistance to make the exercise challenging.

This time you will lie on your side. If you are working your right arm, you will lie down on your left side. Just as with the band version of this exercise, you will bend your elbow at a 90-degree angle and keep your upper arm tucked into your side.

Slowly lift the weight by rotating your arm toward the ceiling while keeping your upper arm against your side. Depending on your strength, your mobility, and the amount of weight you are lifting, you will probably be able to lift the weight until your forearm is pointed toward the ceiling. Again, if you cannot lift that high, that is okay.

Pause at the end of your comfortable range of motion for one second and return to the starting position. Perform this exercise 10-15 times and do 2-3 sets.

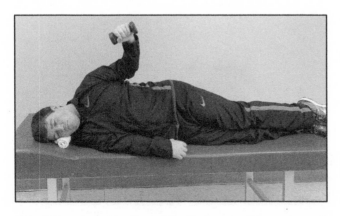

Modification for Band Pull-Apart (Bent Arms)

Exercise 8: Head Nods

This exercise works the muscles that are called the "deep neck flexors." The deep neck flexors are usually thought of as stabilizing muscles of the neck, and they are weak in most people with neck pain.[6] Strengthening these muscles helps reduce neck pain.[7]

Lie on your back with a small towel rolled up and placed under the curve at the back of your neck. Some people lie on the floor to do this exercise, but it is just as effective when lying in bed. While keeping the back of your head in contact with the bed at all times, slowly tuck your chin toward the front of your neck. If you do the exercise correctly, you will make a double chin for a few seconds. It might not be the most flattering look, but it does help with neck pain.

You will feel this exercise deep along the front of your neck and maybe at the back of the neck just below the skull. Hold this for at least 3 seconds, then relax. Repeat 10-15 times and do 2-3 sets.

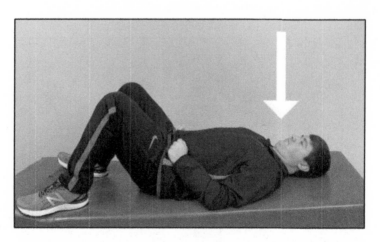

Head Nods

Here is a brief summary of the eight exercises:

1. **Upper Trapezius Stretch**

   - Hold the stretch for 20-30 seconds and repeat 3-5 times

2. **Levator Scapulae Stretch**

   - Hold the stretch for 20-30 seconds and repeat 3-5 times

3. **Pectoralis Major and Minor Stretch**

   - Hold the stretch for 20-30 seconds and repeat 3-5 times

4. **Shoulder Shrugs**

   - Perform 2-3 sets of 10-15 repetitions

5. **Shoulder Blade Squeezes**

   - Perform 2-3 sets of 10-15 repetitions

6. **Band Pull-Apart (Straight Arms)**

   - Perform 2-3 sets of 10-15 repetitions

7. **Band Pull-Apart (Bent Arms)**

   - Perform 2-3 sets of 10-15 repetitions

8. **Head Nods**

   - Perform 2-3 sets of 10-15 repetitions

Foundational Exercises for Neck Pain

That's it! You now have an exercise program for your neck pain. It should take you about 15-20 minutes to finish each day.

If you have neck pain without headaches or arm pain, this program will probably be enough to help you. If you have headaches or arm pain, the next two chapters will give you ideas of exercises that you can add to the eight exercises in this chapter to get even better results!

Don't forget! Access videos of all the exercises in this book by visiting http://bit.ly/NeckExerciseVideos. This will help you ensure that you are performing the exercises correctly!

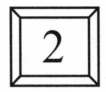

Headache Help

If you have ever suffered with headaches, you know how much they can limit your daily activities. These headaches might keep you from going to the grocery store or even prevent you from playing with your grandkids. Medications might help a little, but you really want to find a way to get rid of your headaches without relying on pills.

The International Headache Society recognizes many different types of headaches,[8] with migraine and tension headaches being the most easily recognized by most people. Another type of headache is a cervicogenic headache. This type of headache comes from some type of dysfunction in the neck, especially the upper part of the neck. This can be decreased movement of one or more joints, tightness of muscles in that region, or a combination of both.

How do you identify a cervicogenic headache? These headaches usually start at the upper part of the neck, near the base of the skull. Pain radiates along one side of the head only and can include the back, side, and front of the head on that side. Many people complain of pain that seems to settle just behind the eye. Cervicogenic headaches are often aggravated by head and neck movement, and firm pressure at the upper part of the neck generally increases the intensity of the headache.[8]

Headache Help

If you have ever been diagnosed with a migraine, you might recognize the familiar pattern of the one-sided headache that settles around the eye. In fact, a recent study found that people with migraines who fail to improve with conventional medical treatment often have problems with their neck also. In these cases, they might have a cervicogenic headache instead of, or in addition to, a migraine headache.[9]

But can you do anything for your headaches other than taking medications? The answer is a resounding yes!

Research has consistently shown that specific exercises are beneficial for patients with cervicogenic headache.[2] These helpful exercises focus on strengthening the deep muscles along the front of the neck and the muscles around the shoulder blades. Sound familiar? That's because these exercises are the same ones listed in Chapter 1. They should be the foundation of the exercise program for your headaches.

The rest of this chapter contains three additional exercises that help many people who have headaches. These exercises are easy to do and require little or no extra equipment for these exercises—just a pillowcase, a towel, and a couple of tennis balls. They are designed to improve the mobility of the upper part of your neck and to reduce the muscle tension in that area.

Headache Help 1: Neck Rotation with Pillowcase

People with cervicogenic headaches usually have limited motion in one or more joints of the upper part of their neck.[10] A physical therapist from New Zealand developed an exercise to improve mobility of this region.[11] A year-long study found that people who use this exercise are able to reduce the severity of their headaches.[12]

To do this exercise, you will need a pillowcase. Start by sitting up straight while looking forward. Feel along the middle of the back of your head, where you will find a part of your skull that sticks out a little more than the rest. From here, move your fingers downward until you find a soft depression. This is where you will place the seam (of the long edge) of your pillowcase.

To improve your ability to turn to the right, grab the left part of the pillowcase with your right hand so that the pillowcase rests against the left side of your face. Use your left hand to grab the right part of the pillowcase so that it rests against the right side of your neck. Turn your head to the right and use your right hand to stretch your neck into slightly more rotation. Hold this stretch for 3 seconds. Repeat for a total of 5 times per side.

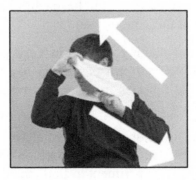

Neck Rotation with Pillowcase

Headache Help 2: Chin Tuck Progression

The purpose of this exercise is to provide a gentle stretch to the muscles of the upper neck, which are often tight in people with headaches. Don't be fooled by the simplicity of this exercise. It has helped many people overcome their headaches.

Take a dish towel and roll it up to 2-3 inches in diameter. Place it under the base of your skull and gently tuck your chin toward the front of your neck without lifting your head. Hold for about 3 seconds and relax.

When you perform this movement, you should notice a slight decrease in the intensity of your headache. Think about your headache on a scale of 0 to 10, with 0 being no pain and 10 being the worst pain ever. You should notice a 1-2 point decrease in your headache with this movement. For example, if your headache is a 6 out of 10 on the pain scale, this movement should reduce the pain to a 4-5 out of 10.

If this movement decreases your headache by 1-2 points, repeat this exercise for a total of 2-3 sets of 10 repetitions. If the movement does not change the severity of your headache or even increases your headache, try one of these modifications:

1. Focus on tucking your chin very gently toward your neck. If you perform a chin tuck too strongly, you might cause the muscles to tighten in response, which could increase your headache.

2. Roll the towel up thicker or smaller. The thickness of the towel can have a big impact on the success of this exercise, so experiment to find the best size for you.

If you try these modifications and it still doesn't help, then you may want to try moist heat or ice for 15 minutes to help with relaxation. Just make sure to place a towel between your skin and the heat or ice. Be careful not to burn your skin. Make sure any redness goes away before repeating the heat or ice.

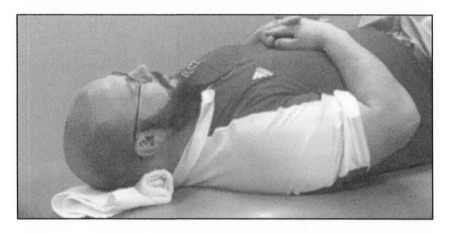

Chin Tuck Progression: Step 1

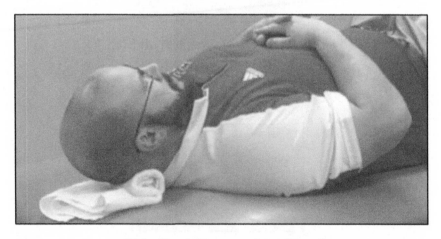

Chin Tuck Progression: Step 2

Headache Help 3: Self-Massage

Like the previous exercise, this one is designed to relax the muscles of the upper neck. This exercise requires slightly more equipment. You will need two tennis balls and some athletic tape. You can find them at a local sporting goods store for $5 to $10.

Before doing the exercise, you will use the two tennis balls and the tape to create a self-massage tool that looks like a peanut. Hold the balls against each other and tape them together by using one strand of tape to encircle the tennis balls (Step 1). Repeat this taping procedure until tape completely surrounds the tennis balls, which usually takes about 4 strands of tape (Step 2).

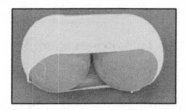

Tennis Ball Self-Massage Tool: Step 1

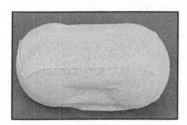

Tennis Ball Self-Massage Tool: Step 2

Now let's talk about how to do the exercise. Lie down on your back either in your bed or on the floor. You will place the tennis balls under your head at the base of your skull. This will place gentle pressure on your neck where the muscles attach to the skull. This gentle, sustained pressure will help your muscles relax.

Lie on the tennis balls for 5-10 minutes to receive the best results. Time will vary per person, and you can do this too long. You might start with 5 minutes first, then add more time if it seems to help. Try this exercise once per day.

This method can be used for pain in the neck, back, shoulder, and any other muscle. You can lean against them with the tennis balls between your body and the bed, floor, or wall. You can also use them to massage muscles by rolling them on your body or gently pressing into pain points and holding for 3-5 minutes.

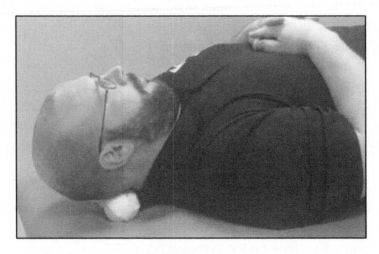

Self-Massage

Headache Help

Here is a brief summary of the three exercises:

1. **Neck Rotation with Pillowcase**
   - Hold the stretch for 3 seconds and repeat 5 times on each side

2. **Chin Tuck Progression**
   - Hold the stretch for 3 seconds and repeat for 2-3 sets of 10 repetitions (20-30 total)

3. **Self-Massage**
   - Lie down in this position for 5-10 minutes once per day

Try these three exercises to help manage your headaches. You might find that one of the exercises doesn't help you. That's okay! Just do the 1-2 exercises that seem to decrease your headaches. Think of these three exercises as options that can help you rather than a strict "prescription" of what you must do.

Also remember to perform the exercises from Chapter 1 in addition to these headache exercises. Those eight "foundational exercises" are vital to long-term improvement of your headaches.

Don't forget! Access videos of all the exercises in this book by visiting http://bit.ly/NeckExerciseVideos. This will help you ensure that you are performing the exercises correctly!

Arm Pain Relief

Many people with neck pain also have pain, numbness, and/or tingling that travels down the arm, sometimes as far as the hand. If you are one of the many people with these symptoms, you know how much they can limit your daily activities. Arm pain tends to be more severe than neck pain, and this can wear you down mentally as much as it does physically.

The combination of neck and arm pain can be caused by multiple structures in the neck and shoulder region. The most common are probably irritated discs, pressure on a nerve, and tight knots in a muscle. While this book cannot cover all the possible causes of arm pain, it covers several exercises to help the most common causes.

So what exercises can help people with neck and arm pain? Unfortunately, this is an area that does not have much high-quality research. Exercises like the "foundational exercises" in Chapter 1 have been successful in the treatment of neck and arm pain, so once again, they should form the core of your exercise program.[13-14] Other exercises, such as the following three exercises used in this chapter, have been used successfully in physical therapy clinics and in research studies as part of a comprehensive treatment plan for people with neck and arm pain.[14-15]

Arm Pain Exercise 1: Seated Chin Tuck

This exercise is very similar to the Head Nod exercise from Chapter 1. Instead of lying on your back, you will sit or stand to perform this exercise. When you do this exercise, you might feel slightly increased neck pain along with decreased arm pain. If this happens, don't be alarmed. It is usually a good sign when pain moves out of the arm, even if your neck pain gets slightly worse.

Sit or stand straight while looking forward. Pull your head straight back without tilting your head up or down. It might help to focus on a spot on the wall while doing this exercise so that your head stays level. Hold this position for 2-3 seconds.

Repeat this exercise 10 times. If it decreases your arm pain, do the exercise as often as you can throughout the day. Aim for once every 30-60 minutes. The key with this exercise is to do it as often as possible. If this exercise increases your arm pain, try it while you are lying on your back. If this helps, do the exercise while lying on your back as often as you can. You probably can't do it every 30-60 minutes if you are working, so just do what you can.

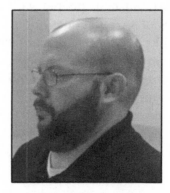

Seated Chin Tuck

Arm Pain Exercise 2: Neck Bend with Pillowcase

When you have pain that radiates from your neck into your arm, it can be very difficult to turn or bend your neck to that side. A physical therapist can often use a hands-on technique to help you turn or bend your neck with less pain. But what about the times when you don't have access to a physical therapist? That is where this exercise becomes very helpful.

Sit or stand straight while looking forward. Using a pillowcase, place the long edge of the pillowcase at the back of the neck where you seem to have the most soreness. Grab each end of the pillowcase with your hands and gently pull forward. While maintaining this forward pull with your hands and the pillowcase, bend your neck toward the painful side.

You should notice that you can move farther and/or with slightly less pain. If not, move the pillowcase slightly up or down on your neck and repeat the movement. This might take several attempts. Just make sure that your motion and pain improve. Hold the position for 2-3 seconds and repeat 10 times. Perform 2-3 sets of this exercise.

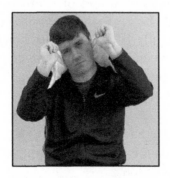

Neck Bend with Pillowcase

Arm Pain Exercise 3: Waiter Drops the Tray

Nerve irritation is a common cause of pain that travels from the neck into the arm. This type of pain is often described as shooting, stabbing, or shocking. It can also cause sensations of burning, tingling, or numbness.

A common way to treat this nerve pain is to perform exercises to gently move the nerve. There are many variations of nerve exercises. Some place tension on the nerve through a series of arm and neck movements. While this can be helpful for specific people with nerve-related arm pain, it can cause further irritation of the nerve in others.

A better way for most people is to perform a series of arm and neck movements that allow the nerve to gently slide as the motions are performed. In this way, you are able to move the nerve in a way that is not painful, helping relieve the nerve pain without causing irritation of the nerve.

Start this exercise by sitting or standing while looking straight ahead. If your right arm is the painful side, raise your right arm so that it's in a position that a waiter or waitress would use to carry a tray. Your arm should be out to the side with your elbow bent. Your elbow should be slightly below shoulder height. In addition, your palm should face the ceiling and your fingers should be pointed to the right. Check the pictures on the next page to make sure that you have the correct starting position.

Likewise, if the pain is in your left arm, your will have your left arm in the waiter's position.

From this position, tilt your head toward the painful side and straighten your elbow. Keep your wrist firm during this movement so that your palm ends up facing toward the right and your fingers are pointed toward the ground. It might help to think about the waiter dropping the tray (while tilting the head toward that side).

Hold this position very briefly (about 1-2 seconds) then reverse the motion to the starting position. Repeat 10 times. If this helps, perform 2-3 sets of the exercise once per day starting the next day.

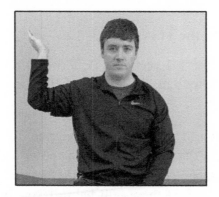

Waiter Drops the Tray: Step 1

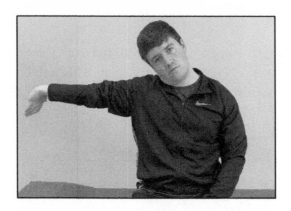

Waiter Drops the Tray: Step 2

Arm Pain Relief

Here is a brief summary of the three exercises:

1. **Seated Chin Tuck**

    • Hold for 2-3 seconds and repeat 10 times. Do this as often as you can during the day.

2. **Neck Bend with Pillowcase**

    • Hold for 2-3 seconds. Perform 2-3 sets of 10 repetitions.

3. **Waiter Drops the Tray**

    • Hold for 1-2 seconds. Perform 10 repetitions the first day. After that, do 2-3 sets of 10.

Getting rid of arm pain can be challenging. It tends to be a slow process. Don't get discouraged! Start with the eight "foundational exercises" from Chapter 1. Then try the three exercises from this chapter. Usually, 2-3 of them will help. If you are having trouble sleeping or working because of arm pain, check out Chapter 5 for helpful tips on managing your pain at home and at work.

Don't forget! Access videos of all the exercises in this book by visiting http://bit.ly/NeckExerciseVideos. This will help you ensure that you are performing the exercises correctly!

Managing Flare-Ups

You know the feeling: You wake up one morning and your neck just doesn't feel right. You try to turn your head to the right, and a sudden jolt of sharp pain stops you from moving even half the amount you can normally turn. Some people call this a "crick in the neck." Whatever you call it, this literal pain in the neck can cause severe pain for several days to several weeks.

What is the cause of this flare-up? It could be from having your neck in an awkward position for a long time (such as when you were sleeping), from performing an activity that made you look up or down for a prolonged period, or from any other number of causes. This temporary "locking up" of your neck can be due to stiffness in one of the joints of your neck, irritation of the capsule that surrounds the joint, or spasm of the nearby muscles. Most likely, it's a combination of two or all three of these reasons.

Regardless of the exact cause, several exercises can be very useful for helping you quickly overcome this temporary setback. These exercises are designed to gently restore motion by allowing neck movement in a way that is much less painful. This encourages your brain to let you move more freely, which will help you overcome the painful and limited movement.

Flare-Up Exercise 1: Multifidus Isometrics

This exercise uses a deep neck muscle, called the multifidus, to help you regain motion. The multifidus is really a series of muscles that span the length of the spine, connecting one bone to the next. This allows the multifidus to precisely control movement of the spine when you move your head, spine, arms, or legs. What makes the multifidus different from most other muscles is that it also attaches into the fibrous capsules of the joints of the spine. As you read on the previous page, sometimes the crick in your neck can be due to irritation or pinching of this capsule. This exercise uses the multifidus muscle to move the joint and capsule in a way that allows the neck to move more freely.

Usually, when you awake with your neck locked up, it will be difficult to look to the right or left and extremely difficult and painful to look up. Sometimes it can be painful to look in both directions, but one way will be worse than the other.

Start this exercise by looking down slightly while sitting. Then place your hand opposite of the painful side behind your head with your palm facing your head. So if you have more trouble turning to the right, you will use your left hand. Push your head gently back into your hand while resisting the movement with your hand. If you do this right, your head will not actually move backward. Hold for 5 seconds. Repeat 3 times. This is the first step.

The second step is slightly different. Place the same hand you used for step one on the side of your head that is the least painful. Push gently into your hand again, holding 5 seconds. Repeat 3 times. Check the motion of your neck again to see if you can move farther and with less pain. You can repeat this exercise multiple times a day.

You should not have sharp pain during this exercise or any numbness, tingling, or burning down your arms afterward. Stop immediately if this makes you worse.

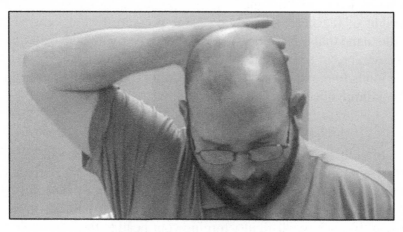

Multifidus Isometrics: Step 1

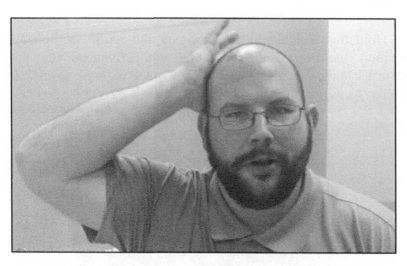

Multifidus Isometrics: Step 2

Flare-Up Exercise 2: Lying Neck Rotation

When you are sitting or standing, the joints of your neck are in what is called a "weight bearing" position. In other words, the weight of the head is applying some pressure to the joints. Now understand that this is normal. However, when you have irritation of one or more of these joints, it can be helpful to take some weight off the joints to regain motion. You can do this by turning your head to the painful side while you are lying down.

Start this exercise while lying on your back in your bed. You can use a small pillow or have your head resting on the bed, depending on which one is more comfortable for you. Perform the exercise by slowly turning your head toward the side that is painful. In other words, if you have difficulty turning your head to the right, you will turn your head to the right during this exercise. Turn as far as you comfortably can. Don't push it too hard. Just perform a gentle motion toward the painful direction.

Hold this position for 2-3 seconds and return to the starting position (looking toward the ceiling while lying on your back). Repeat 10 times and perform 2-3 sets. Do this exercise several times per day as long as it is helping.

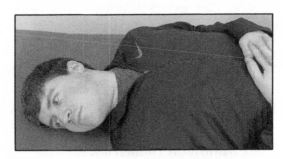

Lying Neck Rotation

Flare-Up Exercise 3: Seated Neck Rotation

In the past, you might have been to a physical therapist or chiropractor who popped your neck. They might have started by rotating or bending your neck in the direction that is less painful. This is because popping your neck toward the non-painful direction increases your ability to turn your neck toward the painful direction.

This exercise uses the same principle. Let's say you have pain with turning your head to the right. Your brain interprets this pain as a threat and causes your muscles to tighten. If you turn your head repeatedly to the left, you are able to do two things. First, you are moving the painful joint slightly, so you are getting some beneficial effects from the movement itself. Second, your brain does not see this movement as a threat, which tends to relax the muscles. The end result is usually increased movement toward the painful direction.

Start by sitting straight while looking forward. Turn your head as far as you can toward the non-painful (or less painful) direction. Hold this position for 2-3 seconds and repeat 10-15 times. Do 2-3 sets before retesting the painful movement. If you can now move farther and/or with less pain, repeat the exercise until you find that it doesn't improve your motion. Try this several times per day.

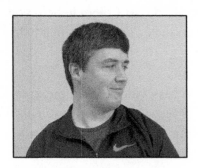

Seated Neck Rotation

Managing Flare-Ups

Here is a brief summary of the three exercises:

1. Multifidus Isometrics

- Push your head backward into your hand and hold for 5 seconds. Repeat 3 times. Then push your head into your hand toward the **non-painful** (or less painful) side. Hold for 5 seconds and repeat 3 times. Do this several times per day.

2. Lying Neck Rotation

- While lying on your back, turn your head toward the **painful** side and hold for 2-3 seconds. Perform 2-3 sets of 10 repetitions. Do this exercise several times per day.

3. Seated Neck Rotation

- While sitting, turn your head toward the **non-painful** side and hold for 2-3 seconds. Repeat for 2-3 sets of 10-15 repetitions. Retest the painful movement. Repeat this sequence until the painful movement doesn't improve.

That's it! These three exercises are great for treating flare-ups of neck pain when you have trouble turning toward one side. As always, if one exercise doesn't seem to help you, don't feel that you have to do it. Just do the 1-2 exercises that help.

Don't forget! Access videos of all the exercises in this book by visiting http://bit.ly/NeckExerciseVideos. This will help you ensure that you are performing the exercises correctly!

Managing Neck Pain at Home and Work

At this point, you have learned how to treat your neck pain, arm pain, and headaches. But is there anything else you can do at home or work to make things even better? Absolutely!

One of the most common complaints in people with neck pain is that they have trouble sleeping because they can't get comfortable. Whether you sleep on your back or on your side, you can do several things to get more restful sleep—which makes all the difference in how you feel the next day! The other common issue that people have is neck pain with sitting, especially when they have to sit for long periods at work. Once again, you have several options that can help you manage your neck pain at home, at work, or during your commute.

The advice on the following pages is helpful for most people. However, you might find that one tip doesn't help you or even makes your pain worse. Here is how to handle those situations. If something does not change your neck pain, try it for several days before deciding that it isn't helpful. Sometimes it takes a while for your body to adapt to something new. If it doesn't help within a week, feel free to stop it. If one of the tips increases your pain, adjust your positioning slightly to see if that helps. If it continues to hurt more, stop it immediately. And if something helps your pain, keep doing it!

Tips for Sleeping on Your Back

First, let's talk about sleeping posture and how to position your neck in bed. This tip will help keep your spine in a more neutral position, which will allow you to sleep better at night. This method of improving sleep is extremely simple to try at home. You don't need any equipment. Just use your pillow and a bath towel. These techniques have helped many people sleep better over the years.

Take a regular bath towel and roll it up long ways. Slip the towel into your pillow case at the bottom of the pillow. Place the pillow back on your bed with the towel on the ceiling side of the pillow. If you have done this correctly, the towel will be pointed in a left-to-right direction rather than pointed from your head to your feet. In this way, the towel will help cradle your neck when you are lying on your back. From here, simply lie back onto the pillow with the towel resting underneath your neck. This will place your neck in a neutral position rather than having it bend forward or backward.

Try to sleep like this for a couple of nights. If you do not see any relief, just go back to sleeping how you were. This is an extremely noninvasive and conservative way of improving sleep.

Along with using a bath towel to support your neck, it's also important to choose a pillow that is the appropriate size. If you are sleeping on your back, you want to use a relatively thin pillow. This is because a thicker pillow often pushes your head forward into an awkward position, which is usually uncomfortable.

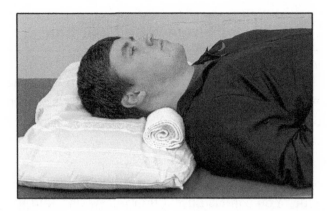

Sleeping on Your Back: Supporting Your Neck

Another thing that helps many people with neck pain sleep more comfortably is to place something under their knees so that their knees are bent. Doing this often feels better for your lower back, which can indirectly help your neck. After all, you are more likely to toss and turn during the night if you are not in a comfortable position for your lower back.

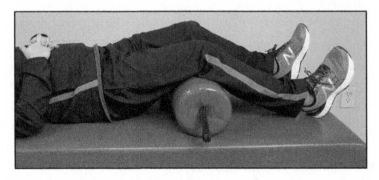

Sleeping on Your Back: Supporting Your Knees and Back

Tips for Sleeping on Your Side

Here is what you do if you are a side sleeper. Keep the towel in the pillow case as described on the previous pages. When you roll over onto either side, the towel will contour to your neck.

It is also helpful to have a thicker pillow if you normally sleep on your side. You can also use a thin pillow and fold it in half so that your pillow is now twice the height. The reason for doing this is that you want to keep your neck in a fairly neutral position, meaning that your neck is not bent toward the bed or toward the ceiling. Since the distance between the side of your head and the outside of your shoulder is fairly large, you will want a thicker pillow to take up this distance and keep your head neutral.

Now that you have your neck in a good position, you will want to address the position of the rest of your body. You want to align the lower areas of your spine to be in a more neutral position. You will do this by positioning your legs and arms with pillows.

First, bring your knees up towards your chest so that your hips and knees are bent in a comfortable position. Then, place a pillow between your knees. Some people find it helpful to fold the pillow so that it is twice as thick, while others prefer placing the pillow so that it runs from the knees all the way to the ankles. Using a pillow between your knees can be helpful for a couple of reasons. It is usually more comfortable because it provides a cushion between the bony parts of your knees. It also keeps your hips and spine in a more neutral position, which typically makes it easier to sleep more soundly through the night.

These changes might be enough for you. If not, consider these other tips on how you can position your arms. To better support your arm that is on top (closer to the ceiling), you can place a pillow or two under this arm so that it rests level with your side. Your body will tell you what is comfortable or not. Just listen to it and add pillows accordingly. To find a better position for your bottom arm, you can move it forward slightly so that you are lying on your shoulder blade more than your shoulder.

Remember that the goal of using these pillows is to help you find a more comfortable sleeping position for your neck. If one of these tips makes you less comfortable, feel free to adjust your position or not follow that particular piece of advice. Also, the goal isn't to sleep with 3-4 pillows for the rest of your life. The purpose is to provide comfort while the exercise program helps you gain control over your neck pain.

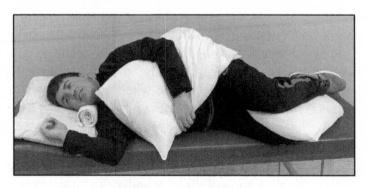

Sleeping on Your Side

Tips for Sitting

The final set of tips in this chapter relates to decreasing neck pain while you are sitting. Before getting to those tips, let's clear up a common myth: There is no single "best" posture. Slouching is not always bad and sitting up straight at all times is not necessary. Your body usually responds best to changing positions multiple times over the course of an hour. With that in mind, let's look at the following tips.

First, it is usually helpful to break of periods of sitting to no longer than 30-60 minutes, especially if you have neck pain. If your job requires sitting for hours at a time, stand up for 1-2 minutes at least every hour. If you are driving for a while, you probably want to take a short break every hour to get out of the car and walk around.

Second, you can help your neck by changing the position of your hips and lower back while you are sitting. Try this experiment. Sit up straight and notice the position of your head and neck. Then round your back into a slouched posture and notice how your head and neck move in response. Usually, they will move forward slightly, which can be uncomfortable when you already have neck pain. If this is the case for you, the next tip will probably help you.

Take two large bath towels and roll them so that they are 2-3 inches thick. Place one towel directly under the bony parts of your buttocks, where you place most of your weight when sitting. By elevating your hips slightly, you will be able to sit in a more upright position with greater ease. Place the other towel in the small of your back against the back support of your chair. This will further support your back and make it easier to sit. Experiment with using just one of these towels or both of the towels and use what feels best.

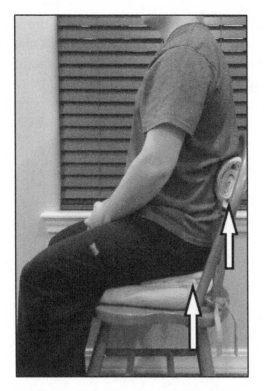

Sitting Position Using Towels

Finally, if you regularly sit at a desk and use a computer, you can make several adjustments to help your neck pain. Use a desk height that allows you to rest your elbows and forearms on the top of the desk without slouching and without shrugging your shoulders. This will help you keep your neck and shoulder muscles relaxed, which will take some stress off your neck. Next, you will probably want to keep the computer directly in front of you. However, experiment with this and see what helps you the most. Some people find it helpful to have their computer slightly to the left or to the right. The important thing is to figure out what works best for you and keep doing it.

Managing Neck Pain at Home and Work

The ideas in this chapter will help you sleep and sit with less neck pain. Remember that these are guidelines that help most, but not all, people with neck pain. Feel free to modify the positions slightly to make your neck more comfortable. In that way, you can customize these recommendations for your own needs.

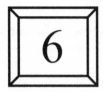

6

Frequently Asked Questions

People have many questions about their neck pain. Some of these questions require a face-to-face consultation to provide specific advice for an individual. However, other questions are more generic and can be answered more easily.

This final chapter answers seven of the most frequently asked questions about neck pain:

1. Is neck pain serious?

2. Does abnormal posture cause neck pain?

3. Is neck pain related to stress?

4. Can neck pain make me dizzy?

5. What about other treatment options for neck pain?

6. Which type of mattress is best for neck pain?

7. Should I get an MRI of my neck?

These answers are not intended as medical advice. Rather, the goal is to deepen your understanding of neck pain. This will help you to ask better questions of your medical provider, which will assist you in making more informed decisions about your health.

Frequently Asked Questions

Is neck pain serious?

Most neck pain is **not** serious. Even if you are having horrible neck pain, it does not mean that it will last a long time, that you will need an MRI, or that it will require surgery. In fact, most cases of neck pain resolve on their own.[16]

Most cases of neck pain are not serious, but what about **your** neck pain? Is there some way to determine when you need to seek medical attention for your neck pain?

Here are a few questions to help determine if you should visit your doctor for your neck pain. If you answer "yes" to any of the following questions, it is a good idea to consult with your doctor.

1. Is your neck pain due to a car wreck or a fall?

2. Is your neck pain getting worse?

3. Do you have pain that radiates into one or both arms?

4. Do you have fever or nausea with your neck pain?

5. Does your neck pain make you feel dizzy?

6. Is your neck pain waking you up at night?

7. Do you have a constant headache that is the worst you have ever experienced?

Answering "yes" to one of these questions does not necessarily mean that your neck pain is serious. However, you should probably consult with your doctor for a full examination. Doctors are skilled at asking questions to determine if your neck pain is serious enough to require additional testing.[17]

46

Does abnormal posture cause neck pain?

Physicians, physical therapists, trainers, and coaches have long argued the reality of "normal posture" and whether or not there is such a thing. Some clinicians even question if "abnormal posture" can cause pain.

While posture is just one of many factors in the development of neck pain, research has shown that postural habits can contribute to your neck pain. Office workers who have neck pain are more likely to work in a posture that involves rounding the upper back and allowing the head to protrude forward.[18] Adolescents who sit for long periods are more likely to have neck pain.[19] Multiple studies have shown an association between neck pain and increased smartphone use.[20-22]

The bottom line is this: Staying in an awkward posture for prolonged periods can lead to (or increase) neck pain. Consider setting up your work area so that you are looking straight ahead toward your computer screen. Keep your computer screen and keyboard at a distance that does not require you to protrude your head and neck forward. When you are talking on the phone while performing another task, avoid the urge to pin the phone between your ear and shoulder so that you can keep your hands free. If your job requires frequent multi-tasking like this, consider getting a headset to avoid this problem.

One last piece of advice: Don't let the words above scare you. Certain postures and movements are not inherently bad. However, it is a good idea to become more aware of the postures or movements that increase your pain. When you understand this, you will know which activities to avoid or reduce until your neck feels better.

Frequently Asked Questions

Is neck pain related to stress?

Almost everyone has heard someone say, "I carry all my stress in my neck and shoulders." You might have even said it yourself.

Research shows a strong relationship between stress and neck pain, especially pain that lasts longer than three months.[23] This is true whether the stress is physical or emotional.[24-26]

When your body is stressed, your muscles are likely to be tense. Imagine you are about to be hit by an oncoming car. What is the first thing you did when you read that sentence? Tense up! That is exactly what you would do if you saw an actual car speeding toward you.

That situation doesn't happen every day, so what about your normal daily activities? A stressful work environment is associated with higher levels of muscle tension and increased neck pain.[27] Constant, low-level stress can worsen neck pain and feelings of muscle tension.

Regardless of the cause of your stress, take some time to relax to see if it helps reduce your neck pain. Some options include getting a massage, taking a walk, or engaging in meditation.

Can neck pain make me dizzy?

Dizziness can be caused by many different conditions, ranging from inner ear problems to more serious conditions such as a stroke.[28] Because of this, it's important to speak with your doctor about your dizziness so that the specific cause can be found and treated.

Dizziness can be related to neck pain, and this condition is called cervicogenic dizziness. This is thought to be uncommon, and the exact cause of cervicogenic dizziness is unknown.[29] The cause could be similar to that of cervicogenic headaches since nerve blocks to the upper part of the neck have been found to improve dizziness.[30] For people with confirmed cervicogenic dizziness, hands-on treatment by a physical therapist improves symptoms at 3 months[31] and 12 months[32] following treatment.

In summary, dizziness can be related to neck pain, although this is an uncommon cause. You should consult with your doctor so that he or she can form an accurate diagnosis. If you have cervicogenic dizziness, you can benefit from seeing a physical therapist who specializes in the treatment of neck pain and dizziness.

What about other treatment options for neck pain?

When self-treatment is not enough to overcome your neck pain, several other options are available, including physical therapy, injections, and surgery. It is important to discuss your specific needs with your doctor. It's also vital that you are educated about these treatment options so that you can make the best decision for your health. Read below for a brief summary of recent research on physical therapy, injections, and surgery for neck pain.

The exercises in this book are based on research into physical therapy for neck pain, arm pain, and headaches. Exercise alone is often enough to eliminate these problems. However, customized treatment by a physical therapist is sometimes needed to help people with neck pain.

Hands-on treatment by a physical therapist, in addition to an exercise program, can provide greater short-term pain relief than exercise alone for people with neck pain and/or headaches.[33] However, long-term improvements are not any greater for those who receive hands-on treatment when compared to those who only perform exercises.[33]

What does this mean for you? First, physical therapy can be very effective for providing short-term pain relief when you need help managing a flare-up of your neck pain. Second, exercises like the ones shown in this book are the most important part of taking control of your neck pain. This is great news! In most cases of neck pain, you are in control of the outcome!

Injections are commonly given to people who have neck pain, especially if they also have arm pain that is radiating from the neck. This is particularly true if someone has tried physical therapy without getting much pain relief. Do these injections work? The most recent research suggests that injections are effective for reducing pain by at least 50% in people with neck and arm pain.[34] In particular, these improvements were found in people with disc herniation, spinal stenosis, or post-surgical pain.

Neck surgery is usually performed after patients with neck pain have been unable to get relief from physical therapy or injections. Again, this is most common in people who have arm pain in addition to their neck pain. For people with neck and arm pain, research suggests that a combination of surgery and physical therapy can provide better relief than physical therapy alone,[35] and these improvements remain 5-8 years later.[36]

Recent advances in neck surgery provide promising results for the treatment of neck and arm pain. When compared to patients who are surgically treated with a fusion, patients who undergo disc replacement surgery generally experience more improvement, and they are less likely to need another neck surgery.[37-39]

Hopefully, this brief review of the research gives you a better idea of other treatment options for your neck. In no way is this intended to take the place of advice from your health care provider. Instead, this research is meant to help you make an informed decision regarding treatment for your neck pain.

Frequently Asked Questions

> ## Which type of mattress is best for neck pain?

Many people have difficulty sleeping because of their neck pain. Some will look for a new mattress in hopes of getting relief. Unfortunately, very little research has examined which mattress is best for people with neck pain. One small study found that a "medium-firm" mattress decreased neck and back pain in older adults when compared to a "high-firm" mattress.[40]

Perhaps a more important question is this: Which pillow is best for neck pain? This was addressed in the previous chapter. However, an additional explanation might clarify the issue.

The main concept to remember is that you generally want to choose a pillow thickness that keeps your head and neck in a neutral alignment. That is, your neck is resting in its natural position instead of being bent forward or to either side.

If you sleep on your side, a thicker pillow is generally more comfortable than a thinner pillow. If you sleep on your back, a thinner pillow will probably feel better. Also remember to use a towel roll in your pillow case as described in the previous chapter.

As with most things, there are exceptions to this rule. If you have neck and/or arm pain that worsens when you look up, you might not be comfortable if you sleep on your back with a thin pillow. A thicker pillow might help decrease neck pain when lying down.

Follow these guidelines for more restful sleep and modify them as needed for your individual needs.

Should I get an MRI of my neck?

Many people with neck pain question why their doctor does not perform an MRI to determine the cause of their pain. Others are frustrated that their insurance refuses to pay for an MRI until they try conservative treatments such as physical therapy. Why do these scenarios occur?

Physicians and insurance companies usually follow standards of care, such as the American College of Radiology Appropriateness Criteria for chronic neck pain.[41] These criteria do not recommend the use of an MRI in most cases of neck pain, unless the patient has neurological signs or symptoms, which might include arm pain, weakness, or decreased reflexes.

Part of the reason why an MRI is not recommended for most people with neck pain is the high likelihood of a "false positive." Simply stated, a false positive is an abnormal finding that is discovered by the MRI but that is not the cause of a patient's symptoms. Research has shown that as many as 90% of people who do not have neck pain have abnormal MRI results![42] Another study has found very little difference when comparing the MRIs of people with neck pain to the MRIs of those without neck pain.[43] Therefore, it can be very difficult to determine if an abnormal finding on MRI is the true cause of someone's neck pain.

For these reasons, most people with neck pain do not need an MRI. As usual, there are always exceptions. Use this information to have an informed discussion with your healthcare provider to determine the best options for your specific case.

OUR FREE GIFT TO YOU

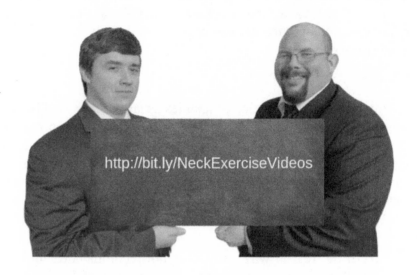

http://bit.ly/NeckExerciseVideos

This book contains many great exercises for people with neck pain. We have provided images and detailed descriptions to help our readers perform the exercises correctly.

We also understand that it can be difficult to learn a new exercise from pictures and text alone. Therefore, we are giving you FREE access to videos of each exercise to help ensure that you are performing the exercises correctly.

To access these videos, visit http://bit.ly/NeckExerciseVideos.

References

1. Kay, Theresa M, et al. "Exercises for Mechanical Neck Disorders." *Cochrane Database of Systematic Reviews*, 2012.

2. Gross, Anita, et al. "Exercises for Mechanical Neck Disorders." *Cochrane Database of Systematic Reviews*, 2015.

3. Medeiros, Diulian M., et al. "Influence of Static Stretching on Hamstring Flexibility in Healthy Young Adults: Systematic Review and Meta-Analysis." *Physiotherapy Theory and Practice*, vol. 32, no. 6, 2016, pp. 438–445.

4. Kruse, Nicholas T., et al. "Influence of Passive Stretch on Muscle Blood Flow, Oxygenation and Central Cardiovascular Responses in Healthy Young Males." *American Journal of Physiology-Heart and Circulatory Physiology*, vol. 310, no. 9, 2016.

5. Kruse, Nicholas T., and Barry W. Scheuermann. "Cardiovascular Responses to Skeletal Muscle Stretching: 'Stretching' the Truth or a New Exercise Paradigm for Cardiovascular Medicine?" *Sports Medicine*, vol. 47, no. 12, May 2017, pp. 2507–2520.

6. Jull, Gwendolen A., et al. "Clinical Assessment of the Deep Cervical Flexor Muscles: The Craniocervical Flexion Test." *Journal of Manipulative and Physiological Therapeutics*, vol. 31, no. 7, 2008, pp. 525–533.

7. Arimi, Somayeh Amiri, et al. "The Effect of Different Exercise Programs on Size and Function of Deep Cervical Flexor Muscles in Patients With Chronic Nonspecific Neck Pain." *American Journal of Physical Medicine & Rehabilitation*, vol. 96, no. 8, 2017, pp. 582–588.

8. "Headache Classification Committee of the International Headache Society (IHS) The International Classification of Headache Disorders, 3rd Edition." *Cephalalgia*, vol. 38, no. 1, 2018, pp. 1–211.

9. Aguila, Maria-Eliza R, et al. "Six-Month Clinical Course and Factors Associated with Non-Improvement in Migraine and Non-Migraine Headaches." *Cephalalgia*, vol. 38, no. 10, 2018, pp. 1672–1686.

10. Hall, T., and K. Robinson. "The Flexion–Rotation Test and Active Cervical Mobility—A Comparative Measurement Study in Cervicogenic Headache." *Manual Therapy*, vol. 9, no. 4, 2004, pp. 197–202.

11. Mulligan, Brian R. *Manual Therapy NAGS, SNAGS, MWMS Etc.* Plane View Services Ltd, 2010.

12. Hall, Toby, et al. "Efficacy of a C1-C2 Self-Sustained Natural Apophyseal Glide (SNAG) in the Management of Cervicogenic Headache." *Journal of Orthopaedic & Sports Physical Therapy*, vol. 37, no. 3, 2007, pp. 100–107.

13. Kuijper, B., et al. "Cervical Collar or Physiotherapy versus Wait and See Policy for Recent Onset Cervical Radiculopathy: Randomised Trial." *Bmj*, vol. 339, July 2009.

14. Diab, Aliaa A, and Ibrahim M Moustafa. "The Efficacy of Forward Head Correction on Nerve Root Function and Pain in Cervical Spondylotic Radiculopathy: a Randomized Trial." *Clinical Rehabilitation*, vol. 26, no. 4, 2011, pp. 351–361.

15. Nee, Robert J., et al. "Neural Tissue Management Provides Immediate Clinically Relevant Benefits without Harmful Effects for Patients with Nerve-Related Neck and Arm Pain: a Randomised Trial." *Journal of Physiotherapy*, vol. 58, no. 1, 2012, pp. 23–31.

16. Vos, Cees J., et al. "Clinical Course and Prognostic Factors in Acute Neck Pain: An Inception Cohort Study in General Practice." *Pain Medicine*, vol. 9, no. 5, 2008, pp. 572–580.

17. Teichtahl, Andrew J., and Geoffrey McColl. "An Approach to Neck Pain for the Family Physician." *Australian Family Physician*, vol. 42, no. 11, 2013, pp. 774-777.

18. Nejati, Parisa, et al. "The Study of Correlation between Forward Head Posture and Neck Pain in Iranian Office Workers." *International Journal of Occupational Medicine and Environmental Health*, Dec. 2015.

19. Prins, Yolandi, et al. "A Systematic Review of Posture and Psychosocial Factors as Contributors to Upper Quadrant Musculoskeletal Pain in Children and Adolescents." *Physiotherapy Theory and Practice*, vol. 24, no. 4, 2008, pp. 221–242.

20. Namwongsa, Suwalee, et al. "Factors Associated with Neck Disorders among University Student Smartphone Users." *Work*, vol. 61, no. 3, May 2018, pp. 367–378.

21. Yang, Shang-Yu, et al. "Association Between Smartphone Use and Musculoskeletal Discomfort in Adolescent Students." *Journal of Community Health*, vol. 42, no. 3, Dec. 2016, pp. 423–430.

22. Xie, Yanfei, et al. "Prevalence and Risk Factors Associated with Musculoskeletal Complaints among Users of Mobile Handheld Devices: A Systematic Review." *Applied Ergonomics*, vol. 59, 2017, pp. 132–142.

23. Ortego, Gorka, et al. "Is There a Relationship between Psychological Stress or Anxiety and Chronic Nonspecific Neck-Arm Pain in Adults? A Systematic Review and Meta-Analysis." *Journal of Psychosomatic Research*, vol. 90, 2016, pp. 70–81.

24. Hannibal, K. E., and M. D. Bishop. "Chronic Stress, Cortisol Dysfunction, and Pain: A Psychoneuroendocrine Rationale for Stress Management in Pain Rehabilitation." *Physical Therapy*, vol. 94, no. 12, 2014, pp. 1816–1825.

25. Sihawong, Rattaporn, et al. "Predictors for Chronic Neck and Low Back Pain in Office Workers: a 1-Year Prospective Cohort Study." *Journal of Occupational Health*, vol. 58, no. 1, 2016, pp. 16–24.

26. Fanavoll, Rannveig, et al. "Psychosocial Work Stress, Leisure Time Physical Exercise and the Risk of Chronic Pain in the Neck/Shoulders: Longitudinal Data from the Norwegian HUNT Study." *International Journal of Occupational Medicine and Environmental Health*, vol. 29, no. 4, Oct. 2016, pp. 585–595.

27. Lundberg, Ulf, et al. "Psychophysiological Stress Responses, Muscle Tension, and Neck and Shoulder Pain among Supermarket Cashiers." *Journal of Occupational Health Psychology*, vol. 4, no. 3, 1999, pp. 245–255.

28. Muncie, Herbert L. "Dizziness: Approach to Evaluation and Management." *American Family Physician*, vol. 95, no. 3, 2017, pp. 154-162.

29. Yacovino, Dario, and Timothy Hain. "Clinical Characteristics of Cervicogenic-Related Dizziness and Vertigo." *Seminars in Neurology*, vol. 33, no. 03, 2013, pp. 244–255.

30. Baron, Eric P., et al. "Role of Greater Occipital Nerve Blocks and Trigger Point Injections for Patients With Dizziness and Headache." *The Neurologist*, vol. 17, no. 6, 2011, pp. 312–317.

31. Reid, S. A., et al. "Comparison of Mulligan Sustained Natural Apophyseal Glides and Maitland Mobilizations for Treatment of Cervicogenic Dizziness: A Randomized Controlled Trial." *Physical Therapy*, vol. 94, no. 4, Dec. 2013, pp. 466–476.

32. Reid, Susan A., et al. "Manual Therapy for Cervicogenic Dizziness: Long-Term Outcomes of a Randomised Trial." *Manual Therapy*, vol. 20, no. 1, 2015, pp. 148–156.

33. Miller, Jordan, et al. "Manual Therapy and Exercise for Neck Pain: A Systematic Review." *Manual Therapy*, vol. 15, no. 4, 2010, pp. 334–354.

34. Manchikanti, Laxmaiah. "Do Cervical Epidural Injections Provide Long-Term Relief in Neck And Upper Extremity Pain? A Systematic Review." *Journal of Spine*, vol. 03, no. 05, 2014.

35. Engquist, Markus, et al. "Surgery Versus Nonsurgical Treatment of Cervical Radiculopathy." *Spine*, vol. 38, no. 20, 2013, pp. 1715–1722.

36. Engquist, Markus, et al. "A 5- To 8-Year Randomized Study on the Treatment of Cervical Radiculopathy: Anterior Cervical Decompression and Fusion plus Physiotherapy versus Physiotherapy Alone." *Journal of Neurosurgery: Spine*, 2017, pp. 19–27.

37. Rao, Min-Jie, et al. "Cervical Disc Arthroplasty versus Anterior Cervical Discectomy and Fusion for Treatment of Symptomatic Cervical Disc Disease: a Meta-Analysis of Randomized Controlled Trials." *Archives of Orthopaedic and Trauma Surgery*, vol. 135, no. 1, May 2014, pp. 19–28.

38. Zhu, Yuhang, et al. "Cervical Disc Arthroplasty Versus Anterior Cervical Discectomy and Fusion for Incidence of Symptomatic Adjacent Segment Disease." *Spine*, vol. 41, no. 19, 2016, pp. 1493–1502.

39. Hu, Yan, et al. "Mid- to Long-Term Outcomes of Cervical Disc Arthroplasty versus Anterior Cervical Discectomy and Fusion for Treatment of Symptomatic Cervical Disc Disease: A Systematic Review and Meta-Analysis of Eight Prospective Randomized Controlled Trials." *Plos One*, vol. 11, no. 2, Dec. 2016.

40. Ancuelle, Victor, et al. "Effects of an Adapted Mattress in Musculoskeletal Pain and Sleep Quality in Institutionalized Elders." *Sleep Science*, vol. 8, no. 3, 2015, pp. 115–120.

41. Daffner, Richard H. "Radiologic Evaluation of Chronic Neck Pain." *American Family Physician*, vo. 82, no. 2, 2010, pp. 959-964.

42. Matsumoto, Morio, et al. "Age-Related Changes of Thoracic and Cervical Intervertebral Discs in Asymptomatic Subjects." *Spine*, vol. 35, no. 14, 2010, pp. 1359–1364.

43. Siivola, Sari M., et al. "MRI Changes of Cervical Spine in Asymptomatic and Symptomatic Young Adults." *European Spine Journal*, vol. 11, no. 4, Sept. 2002, pp. 358–363.

ABOUT THE AUTHORS

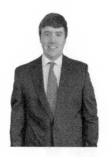

Mark Green graduated with his Doctor of Physical Therapy degree from Louisiana State University Health Sciences Center in Shreveport, LA in 2009. He became board-certified in orthopedic physical therapy in 2012. He is the owner of Sports Orthopedic and Spine Therapy of Louisiana, where his mission is to help patients return to the activities they love without having to rely on medications or surgery.

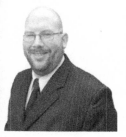

Jeremy Sutton graduated with his Doctor of Physical Therapy degree from The University of St. Augustine for Health Sciences in St. Augustine, FL in 2009. He is the owner of Servant PT of Louisiana, and the creator and host of the Servant PT Podcast. His mission is to truly serve his patients and anyone else who needs life-changing improvements through education and motivation.

OUR FREE GIFT TO YOU

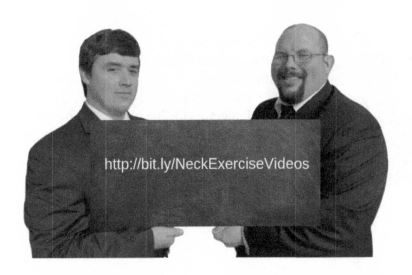

http://bit.ly/NeckExerciseVideos

This book contains many great exercises for people with neck pain. We have provided images and detailed descriptions to help our readers perform the exercises correctly.

We also understand that it can be difficult to learn a new exercise from pictures and text alone. Therefore, we are giving you FREE access to videos of each exercise to help ensure that you are performing the exercises correctly.

To access these videos, visit http://bit.ly/NeckExerciseVideos.